Vita-Guard Weight Loss

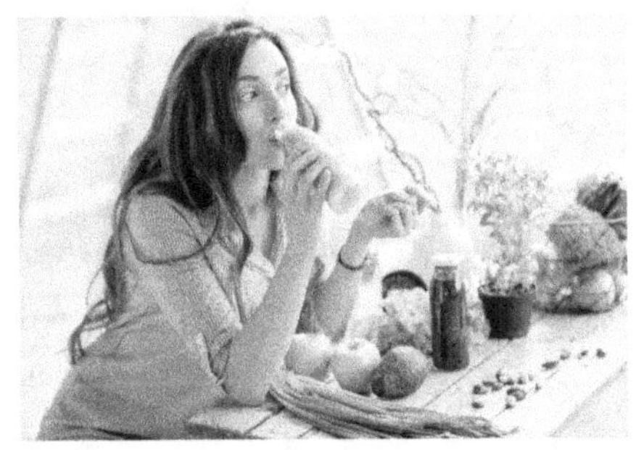

Raymond E. Smith

Published by

Sanway International
91 E. Main Street
Inman, SC 29349

Email: vitaguard1912@gmail.com

Dedicated to

Everyone who is over weight. My hope is that all of you get tremendous results from reading this book.

Table of Contents

Chapter One

Dangers of Over weight

Carrying around too much weight feels uncomfortable, and it can also damage your health. According the Centers of Disease Control and Prevention (CDC), obesity rates have skyrocketed in the United States in recent years. As of 2010, more than one-third of American adults were considered obese.

One method that can help a person lose weight is to limit the number of calories taken in through their diet. The other way is to burn extra calories with exercise.

Avoid fad diet programs. They are only temporary. The best way to get permanent weight loss is by changing your life style.

Dangers of Heart Disease

Changing your life style includes getting a proper amount of food, exercise and getting mentally fit. This book is going to cover all these requirements to permanently lose weight.

Your weight and your risk for heart disease are connected. But that doesn't mean being overweight guarantees that you'll have heart problems. There are ways to reduce your risk for a cardiac event and weight loss may be one of them. But first it's important to learn the facts about heart disease and weight loss.

What Is Heart Disease?

Heart disease is a number of abnormal conditions that affect the heart and the blood vessels in the heart. There are many different types of heart disease, but common forms include coronary artery disease, heart failure, and arrhythmia. The most common form of heart disease is coronary artery disease, a narrowing or blockage of coronary arteries, which is the major reason people have heart attacks.

Heart Disease Facts and Figures

According to the American Heart Association statistics compiled in 2018, cardiovascular disease accounts for nearly 836,546 deaths or about 1 of every 3 deaths in the US. It remains the leading cause of death in this country. Roughly 2,300 Americans die of cardiovascular disease each day, an average of 1 death every 38 seconds.

Approximately every 40 seconds, an American will have a heart attack. The average age for a first heart attack is 65.6 years for males and 72.0 years for females.

The report also notes that someone in the US has a stroke about once every 40 seconds. Stroke accounts for one out of every 19 deaths in the US each year.

About 92.1 million American adults are currently living with some form of either cardiovascular disease or after-effects of a stroke. Nearly half of all black adults have some form of cardiovascular disease, 47.7 percent of females and 46.0 percent of males.

The Heart Disease and Weight Loss

Heart disease and weight loss are closely linked because your risk for heart disease is associated with your weight. If you are overweight or obese, you may be at higher risk for the condition.

Medical experts consider obesity and being overweight to be a major risk factor for both coronary heart disease and heart attack. Being 20 percent overweight or more significantly increases your risk for developing heart disease, especially if you have a lot of abdominal fat. The American Heart Association has found that even if you have no other related health conditions, obesity itself increases risk of heart disease.

Being sedentary also causes your heart disease risk to increase. A sedentary lifestyle may be more dangerous for women. Inactive females are more likely to become diabetic, have high blood pressure and high cholesterol. All three of these conditions increase the chance of developing heart disease.

Other over weight problems

Obesity can lead to a number of serious health problems, other than the heart such as; diabetes, stroke, and some types of cancer. If you are over weight, by all means get some help.

Being sedentary also causes your heart disease risk to increase. A sedentary lifestyle may be more dangerous for women. Inactive females are more likely to become diabetic, have high blood pressure and high cholesterol. All three of these conditions increase the chance of developing heart disease.

Other over weight problems

Obesity can lead to a number of serious health problems, other than the heart such as; diabetes, stroke, and some types of cancer. If you are over weight, by all means get some help.

Eating the Right Foods

Losing weight starts in the kitchen, and what you eat is far more important than how you exercise because weight loss is 70% what you eat and 30% exercise. You can exercise daily and not see the scale move if your diet is not right.

Top Foods that Burn Fat:

- Hot Peppers

- Green Tea and Coffee

- Whole Grains, Quinoa and Oats

- Grapefruit and other Citrus Fruits

- Lean Poultry and Fish

- Beans and Lentils

- Berries

- Apples

- Almonds, Almond milk and Almond butter

- Eggs

- Greek Yogurt

- Spinach and Broccoli

Steps to Help You Lose Weight

1. Remove all processed foods and artificial sweeteners from your diet.
2. Plan your meals and log what you eat and drink.
3. Move your body more. Walk more every day
4. Drink a gallon of water a day.
5. Clean out your cabinets and refrigerator. Get rid of things that are against your weight loss plan. If you don't have it you can't eat it.
6. Take your Vita-Guard vitamins every day.
7. If possible listen to a hypnosis CD every day.
8. Get plenty sleep.

Exercise

Combining exercise with a healthy diet is a more effective way to lose weight than depending on calorie restriction alone. Exercise can prevent or even reverse the effects of certain diseases. Exercise lowers blood pressure and cholesterol, which may prevent a heart attack.

In addition, if you exercise, you lower your risk of developing certain types of cancers such as colon and breast cancer. Exercise is also known to help contribute to a sense of confidence and well-being, thus possibly lowering rates of anxiety and depression.

Exercise is helpful for weight loss and maintaining weight loss. Exercise can increase metabolism, or how many calories you burn in a day. It can also help you maintain and increase lean body mass, which also helps increase number of calories you burn each day.

How much exercise is needed?

To reap the health benefits of exercise, it is recommended that you to perform some form of aerobic exercise at least three times a week for a minimum of 20 minutes per session. However, more than 20 minutes is better if you want to actually lose weight. Incorporating just 15 minutes of moderate exercise — such as walking one mile — on a daily basis will burn up to 100 extra calories (assuming you don't consume excess calories in your diet afterwards). Burning 700 calories a week can equals 10 lbs. of weight loss over the course of a year.

Aerobic

No matter what exercise program you implement, it should include some form of aerobic or cardiovascular exercise. Aerobic exercises get your heart rate up and your blood pumping. Aerobic exercises may include walking, jogging, cycling, swimming, and dancing. You can also work out on a fitness machine such as a treadmill, elliptical, or stair stepper

Change your life style

The total amount of exercise you engage in during a day matters more than whether or not you do it in a single session. That's why small changes in your daily routine can make a big difference in your waistline.

Healthy lifestyle habits to consider include:

Walking or riding your bike to work or while running errands.

Taking the stairs instead of the elevator

Parking farther away from destinations and walking the remaining distance

Remember: If you keep doing what you have always done, and you will be what you've al ways been.

Personal note: I had gained 38 lbs. It hurt to bend over and tie my shoes. I was completely miserable. I decided I had to lost the extra weight. When I carried my wife to the mall, I would walk the circumference of the parking lot while she shopped. When I went to an office building or the hospital for a visit, I walked the stairs rather than ride the elevator. In a short while I lost the 38 lbs.

Activities	Calories Burned
Playing baseball, golf, or cleaning the house	240 to 300
Brisk Walking, biking, dancing, or gardening	370 to 460
Playing football, jogging at nine-mile a minute pace or swimming	580 to 730
Skiing, racquetball, or running at seven-minute mile pace	740 to 920

Talk to your doctor before you start a new exercise program, especially if you are planning on doing vigorous exercise. This is especially important if you have:

- heart disease

- lung disease

- diabetes

- kidney disease

- arthritis

People who have been very inactive for the recent months, who are overweight, or have recently quit smoking should also talk to their doctors before staring a new exercise program.

When you are first starting a new exercise

program, it's important to pay attention to the signals your body is giving you. You should push yourself so that your fitness level improves. However, pushing yourself too hard can cause you to injure yourself. Stop exercising if you start to experience pain or shortness of breath.

Get Accountability and Support

Many apps can help you track your eating. Since you probably have your smartphone with you all the time, you can use it to keep up with your plan. Or keep a pen-and-paper food journal of what you ate and when.

Hundreds of fad diets, weight-loss programs and outright scams promise quick and easy weight loss. However, the foundation of successful weight loss remains a healthy, calorie-controlled diet combined with increased physical activity. For successful, long-term weight loss, you must make permanent changes in your lifestyle and health habits.

How do you make those permanent changes? Consider following these six strategies for weight-loss success.

Make a commitment

Long-term weight loss takes time and effort — and a long-term commitment. Make sure that you're ready to make permanent changes and that you do so for the right reasons.

To stay committed to your weight loss, you need to be focused. It takes a lot of mental and physical energy to change your habits.

So as you're planning new weight-loss-related lifestyle changes, make a plan to address other stresses in your life first, such as financial problems or relationship conflicts. While these stresses may never go away completely, managing them better should improve your ability to focus on achieving a healthier lifestyle. Once you're ready to launch your weight-loss plan, set a start date and then — start.

or relationship conflicts. While these stresses may never go away completely, managing them better should improve your ability to focus on achieving a healthier lifestyle. Once you're ready to launch your weight-loss plan, set a start date and then — start.

Find your inner motivation

No one else can make you lose weight. You must undertake diet and exercise changes to please yourself. What's going to give you the burning drive to stick to your weight-loss plan?

Make a list of what's important to you to help stay motivated and focused, whether it's an upcoming beach vacation or better overall health. Then find a way to make sure that you can call on your motivational factors during moments of temptation. Perhaps you want to post an encouraging note to yourself on the pantry door, for instance.

While you have to take responsibility for your own behavior for successful weight loss, it helps to have support — of the right kind. Pick people to support you who will encourage you in positive ways, without shame, embarrassment or sabotage.

Ideally, find people who will listen to your

concerns and feelings, spend time exercising with you or creating healthy menus, and who will share the priority you've placed on developing a healthier lifestyle. Your support group can also offer accountability, which can be a strong motivation to stick to your weight-loss goals.

If you prefer to keep your weight-loss plans private, be accountable to yourself by having regular weigh-ins, recording your diet and exercise progress in a journal, or tracking your progress using digital tools.

Enjoy healthier foods

Adopting a new eating style that promotes weight loss must include lowering your total calorie intake. But decreasing calories need not mean giving up taste, satisfaction or even ease of meal preparation.

One way you can lower your calorie intake is by eating more plant-based foods — fruits, vegetables and whole grains. Strive for variety to help you achieve your goals without giving up taste or nutrition.

Conditioning Your mind

Before you can make worthwhile improvements including losing weight you need to condition your mind.

In the following pages we are going to lead you through the process of mind conditioning. Regardless, if you want to lose weight or build an empire the rest of this book is necessary.

Please read carefully. Weight loss is not a casual thing to do, it takes a sincere effort with the proper attitudes.

Chapter Two
Getting Ready For Change

One cannot change anything until they are ready. You also cannot change anything about yourself until you recognize the need for change.

Getting ready for change is simple, but certain steps must be followed. You cannot eliminate these steps and expect to change your life.

Step one: Examine yourself carefully. What do you want to change? Why do you want it changed? Do some soul searching. Fully understand these two questions. Do you want to change? ...

Basically, you want to lose weight, have a healthier body and look attractive.

Napoleon Hill said, "You can accomplish anything that you can imagine." If you can get a clear picture of what you want, you have the ability to make it happen.

Before continuing let's look at the word "Success."

What is Success?

Some say winning the lottery. Others say getting what I want. Let me give you a definition that you need to memorize. *Success is a state of mind induced by the setting and accomplishing of goals which are both meaningful and objective.*

Success is the journey, not the destination. Success is when you take big goals and break them down into little goals and accomplish a little each day. If success was a the end of the rainbow you would spend a miserable life getting there.

Success has nothing to do with the size of your bank account, the home you live in or the kind of car you drive.

Success is an attitude. "It's not your aptitude, but your attitude that determines your altitude." "Life has many ups and downs, but your attitude when you are down will determine how high you will go when you are up." An attitude is how you feel about something.

Attitudes can be changed very quickly. Someone tells you, You have a bad attitude." You answer, "I know but I can't change."

Let me tell you how quickly you can change your attitude. Scenario: You have a bad day at work. Coming home you have a flat tire and ruined your best shirt. When you get home your wife meets you at the door with a handful of bills. You get to the dinner table and someone spills a glass of milk and it runs into your lap. About that time the phone rings. With frustration you answer, "WHAT?" Within a few seconds you say in a mellow voice, "Oh I didn't know it was you mother." See how quickly you can change.

Chapter Three

Making Your Goals

You may be thinking I already have a goal. I know what I want. A goal is more than a Santa Clause list. Knowing what you want is just part of a goal. Goals have three parts; <u>what</u>, <u>when</u> and <u>how</u>. Without all three parts you may never achieve what you want.

Let's take it apart and look at one at a time.

WHAT: What do you want? Pin it down to your most wanted. What is your number one goal? Think about it carefully. What do you want more than anything else? Get your priorities in order.

It may be more money, a new home, a promotion at work, a new car, a boat, etc. It's your decision.

Don't let family or friends influence your decision, or to lose weight. Your goal is personal.

WHEN: When do you want it? Someone said, "Some day I'm gonna make a lotta money." That person may never accomplish anything worthwhile because Some day is not on the calendar. Gonna is not is the dictionary. Lotta can not be rung up on a cash register. Set a definite date. Keep in mind permanent weight loss should be two lbs. per week.

HOW: What are you going to do to get what you want? This step is really important. Remember anything you can imagine you can accomplish. For you to lose weight you need to Eat right, take your Vita-Guard and exercise.

I worked for Spartan Food Systems for four years and built 23 stores.

My last store with Spartan Food System was in Athens, Alabama. There were some challenging moments during the finish of the job, that were frustrating. It was time for the light fixtures to be delivered, but they didn't come. I called the lighting supplier and he said, "The fixtures you are using are manufacturer in Italy and we are out of them." He went on to say, "The job in Mississippi has some left over, I will call and have them delivered to you." I thanked him for his help.

After five days, the fixtures didn't come. I called the supplier again, "Where are my fixtures," I asked? "Raymond, I am sorry, they made a mistake and sent the fixtures back here to the warehouse. I will get them on the next truck coming your way and you should have them in about five days." I was getting hot under the collar, but tried to stay calm. "That's not good enough this job is schedule to finish in three days. I have never been late with a job and I won't be late with this one," I told him.

The manager of the lighting company saw

that I was determined. He said, "Can you meet the truck half way, if I send them on our truck?" "Yes, I can," I told him. "Okay, meet the truck at the intersection of I-85 and 285, in Atlanta, at 10:00 tomorrow morning," He instructed me.

I was apprehensive about driving to Atlanta. I had already worked two days and a night, without sleep. After working that many hours, straight, without sleep, on another job, I laid down on a stack of sheetrock and dozed off. When I awoke, one of the laborers said, "Boss, we thought you were dead."

Even with a lack of rest, to keep my reputation, I was willing to make the four hour trip.

At 10:00, I was sitting in a Waffle House, drinking coffee, waiting for the truck. Shortly, I saw the one-ton stake body truck with the company's name on it. I also saw, there were no light fixtures on the truck. The driver made the clover leaf circle and pulled into the Waffle House parking lot. I yelled at the driver, "Where are my light fixtures?" The driver looking surprised said, "The boss didn't say anything about any light fixtures. He just said gas up the truck and meet you here."

I was fit to be tied. I got on the phone with the manager and said, "WHAT HAPPENED TO MY LIGHT FIXTURES?" The manager very apologetically said, "I have already discovered the problem. Since it's my fault if you will stay where you are, I will put the fixtures in my station wagon and bring them to you personally." I agreed. What else could I do? Late that afternoon, I got back to the job and the electrician finished his part of the contract. The job was completed on time.

What are you going to do to reach your goal? Write out a plan of action.

Setting a target date for your goal.

There are three time spans for target dates.

Short range; up to six months. Medium range; six months to two years, Long range; more than two years.

Write your goals on paper. "Writing crystallizes thought and thought provokes action." Let's say your goal is to lose 10 lbs. in the next month. (That's what you want.) You want it in one month. (That's when you want it.) You will get it by sticking to your diet, exercising and taking your Vita-Guard every day. (That's how you will get it.)

Goals must to be specific. If your goal does not specify the model, make and color of the car of car and you walk onto the car lot not knowing exactly what you want the salesman will sell you what he wants to sell. That's his goal.

Definite goals are like a train, it gives you a track to run on, or like a ship, a rudder to guide you on the stormy seas, they help you to get where you want to go.

Once you have set your goals and written them down you are ready for the next step.

Chapter Four

Get Motivated

*"Nothing Happens Until Someone
is Motivated."*

Motivation is that which causes action. There are three basic kinds of motivation.

Motivation is generally defined as the force that compels us to action. It drives us to work hard and pushes us to succeed. Motivation influences our behavior and our ability to accomplish goals.

There are many different forms of motivation. Each one influences behavior in its own unique way. No single type of motivation works for everyone.

People's personalities vary and so accordingly does the type of motivation, that is most effective at inspiring their conduct.

Incentive Motivation: This type of motivation requires a hunger for what you want. It's like tying a carrot in front of a donkey and if his is hungry he will try to get the carrot and pull the cart.

Let's say you eat a big breakfast of ham, eggs and biscuits. A few minutes later someone ask you to eat. You will probably turn it down because there is not a hunger for food.

There are a many different reasons why we do things. Sometimes we are motivated to act because of internal desires and wishes, but at other times our behaviors are driven by a desire for external rewards. The incentive theory is one of the major theories of motivation and suggests that behavior is motivated by a desire for reinforcement or incentives.

Sales companies offer incentives to the sales force in order to get them to work harder.

Fear Motivation: Fear is the worse kind of motivation. It destroys imitative. This is when you whip the donkey to make him run.

At work the boss says, "Get the job done or else." Or, something worse. He is using fear motivation to increase production.

This is the saddest of all motivational factors. Fear of rejection, fear of loss of respect, loss of money and country club status. It's related to the above motivations, but from a different perspective. People who are motivated by fear are motivated from a position of having made it and are afraid of losing it. Its real difference is in its motivational power.

Fear motivation involves punishment or negative consequences. This type of motivation is commonly used to motivate students in the education system and also frequently in a professional setting to motivate employees. If we break the rules or fail to achieve the set goal, we are penalized in some way.

Attitude Motivation: This is when you convince the donkey that he is a race horse and he will run because he wants to run.

Attitude motivation is about how people think and feel. "It is their confidence, their belief in themselves, their attitude to life – be it positive or negative. It is how they feel about the future and how they react to the past.

Many want to lose weight. Every person needs to know that they are important and "they matter". People wish to be treated well, feel valued and respected, be proud of the place they work, and get satisfaction from what they're contributing.

Think about how can you motivate and inspire people by valuing them and recognizing their contribution if you wish to see the amazing value of just making someone feel important and loved.

A change in attitude is changing how you feel. Change how you see things. The world around you looks different.

"Silicon Valley innovators have uniquely learned how to define, design, and deliver innovation with a massive degree of flexibility and concurrency." ~ Christopher Meyer

Chapter Five

Build An Obsession

When you know what you want, you have written your goals, you are motivated; now it's time to build an obsession.

Obsession is described as a burning desire. One can have a casual desire which is no more than a list of "It would be nice to do it." Your goals must become an obsession.

Obsession is the ingredient that burns the path to success. W. Clement Stone lived an obsessed life. At a young age he was an agent for his mother's insurance company. He had a burning desire to own his own company.

Stone searched for a company that was licensed in several states. Months went by with no avail. He kept searching. He put the word out in the industry. Finally, he learned that Pennsylvania Casualty Company was for sale. It had all the requirements to meet his goal.

Stone met with the principals of the company. He had very little cash to pay for the company. He was relying on negotiating a plan when he got there. Much like today's Donald Trump.

They ask Stone how he intended to pay for the company. He answered, "You own Commercial Credit. I will borrow the money from your company to pay for it." He borrowed $1,600,000.00 and closed the deal in one day.

Today the company is known as Combined Insurance Company. I have personally had a policy with them for about 10 years.

When you approach something with an obsession others can see the fire burning within you.

All obsessions are not good. Ted Bundy, the rapist and serial killer was on trial in 1978, told

James Dobson that reading police magazines and pornography made his life obsessed to what he did.

Important: Everything we see, hear, feel, touch or taste goes into our sub-conscious mind and influences our life. Build the right obsession by guarding what your mind is exposed. Read the right materials. Listen only to what is beneficial to your obsession.

With today's technology you can read and listen to CDs where ever you go. My friend, Dr, Mack Douglas said, "You can turn your car into a university." We spend hours a week driving, sometimes suck in traffic when we could be listening to positive messages. Suggestion to build an obsession:

(1) Write your goals on paper. Follow the suggestions in chapter two. This is imperative. I hope you have already taken the time to do this.

(2) Write a plan for attaining your goal. You may have already done this in short sketchy state-

ments. Here go into details.

(3) Read your statement aloud several times a day. Start your day with reading your goals and plan for attainment. Read as often during the day as possible. Most important read it just before going to sleep at night. Everyone, without exception, go into hypnosis seconds before they go to sleep. This allows your sub-conscious to work on the goal while you are sleeping. This is where the statement, "Let me sleep on it." comes from.

After a while you will memorize your goals. This allows you to repeat it more often. Do it while you drive, while you work, and while you do most anything.

(4) Gather clippings to remind you of your goal. If your goal is to buy a new Buick; go to your dealer and get the largest picture you can of the exact car and color you want. Make a scrape book. Place some clipping where you will see it most often;

on your sun visor, refrigerator, mirror, etc. Larry Grizzell, a motivator carries a silver dollar to remind him of the money he intends to earn.

A motivation to lose weight may be pictures of new clothes or anything you would like to do but right now you are unable to do because you are over weight.

(5) Spend some time each day visualizing your goal. Some may call this day-dreaming but it is an important step to accomplishing your goals. The mind does not read words, it reads pictures. Boost your minds ability by translating the words into pictures. Visualize your self as being thin and health. Whatever your goal is create it into pictures.

(6) Expect results. The power of expectation may be one of the greatest powers we have. We have to expect something to happen to make it so.

(7) Use self motivators. Some use, "I feel

health, I feel happy, I feel fantastic" to start their day. You cold say, "Every day in every way I am getting thinner and thinner." Try this and see the wonderful affect it has on your life.

Create your own self-motivators in relation to your goal. Use these to ignite a fire for your goals.

Chapter Six

Create a Sincere Enthusiasm

*"Enthusiasm is an outward expression
of an inward feeling."*

Real enthusiasm comes from within. Fake enthusiasm can be detected easily. Although, igniters can be used to build your enthusiasm.

Think about a hay stack. You can tell it to burn and it doesn't. If you use a match for an igniter it will burn. It's like priming a pump before you can get water. One of the popular lines used by Zig Ziglar, he and his friend stopped along the road in Alabama to get some water. His friend pumped several times and did not get water. Zig said, "Jimmy you have to prime the pump." While on a motivational tour I met the Jimmy that was with Zig.

One way to prime the pump is to associate with people who are already excited. In 1976, I was living in Charlotte, NC. This was during a very deep recession. I was out of work and on the verge of becoming depressed. I didn't want that to happen. I looked in the newspaper to see what was going on around town that was free.

There was an Amway rally at the auditorium starting in a few minutes. I told my wife, "Let's go and see who is speaking. When we got there it had already started. We could hear the excitement long before we got in the door. Every seat in auditorium was filled and hundreds standing. We pushed our way through the crowd and to our surprise Pat Boone was the key speaker.

The place was really rocking. We stood and heard the rest of the speakers for the night. We left highly enthused and excited.

You can go to meetings like this, with no intention of getting involved with their program, but to ignite your enthusiasm.

Dale Carnegie, Frank Bettger, W. Clement Stone and Napoleon Hill all teach that if you act enthusiastic you will become enthusiastic. Ira Hayes who was with the National Cash Register Company said, "We have to condition our minds before we can become enthusiastic."

How do we condition our minds for enthusiasm? Start by getting organized. This mean organize everything in your life. Start with your desk. A disorganized desk can confuse your mind. Organize you schedule. Organize your work, your leisure time, your room and everything.

When your life is not organized artificial stimulus has a short range effect. I have seen sales meeting at 9:00 in the morning where they clapped their hands, sang a song and did all the artificial stimulus and by 2:00 those who were not organized ran out of steam. But, those who were organized had enthusiasm for the rest of the day and were productive.

The story was told about National Cash Register Company in the early days when many merchants were still using a cigar box to keep their money. The sales director called all the sales force to come to Chicago for a convention. He wanted to introduce a modern cash register. The first day the listened to all the advantages of this new machine.

The next morning they assembled and one by one started complaining, "Our merchants will not pay that much money for a box to keep their cash when the cigar box is free." They had no enthusiasm for selling the product. After listening to their complaints he instructed the tour guide to take them to another part of the city and spend the entire day.

He called in a wrecking company and demolished the building and a landscaping company to plant sod and trees. When they arrived the next morning they were shocked that everything was different. The sales director stood before them and said, "Gentlemen anything you want in life can be done." He dismissed them to go home. Sales were outstanding from what they earlier said was impossible.

Maintain a savings account. I have a desk plate that says, "Part of all I earn is mine to keep." I recommend that you read the story of the richest man in Babylon. The book reveals how to keep 10% of all your earning for yourself. This will help you to build your real enthusiasm.

Promote yourself on social networks such as Facebook, Tweeter, Pinterest and others. Keep your friends informed of your activities. Please avoid useless posting of what you eat, how long you slept or what you dog likes to do. Keep it positive for a professional image.

Make firm decisions. Many people have trouble making decisions. Henry Ford was know for making quick decisions and slow for changing his mind.

The story was told about a lady who went to a psychiatrist. She said, "My life is constantly making decisions. I make thousands of decisions every day." He asked, "What kind of work do you do." She said, "I work in a orange juice plant and I have to decide which oranges are good or bad." Life is filled with decision making. Learn to make firm decisions on things that matter.

How to make firm decisions.

(1) Clearly state the problem. Many times we have problems and don't understand what the problem is. A clearly stated problem is half solved.

(2) Gather more information. Sometimes deci-

sions can't be made because we don't have enough information. When you have all the information you might use the Ben Franklin method for making the decision.

Take a sheet of paper and list the pros and the cons. Draw a line down the center of the paper. On one side list the pros and the other side list the cons. Give each item a score of I to 10 based on the priority or importance of the item. When you are finished total your score. This will make the decision much easier.

(3) Be a leader. Volunteer to work with groups or committees. Leaders are not born. I have seen baby boys and baby girls but I have never seen a new born leader. Leadership must be developed. Leaders stand head and shoulders above the crowd.

Chapter Seven

Develop Confidence

Confidence and faith are two of the most important attributes to obtaining your goal. They have to be acquired.

Faith is believing we will receive the things we hope for. When we hope for something we must have complete assurance that we will get what we hoped for. A lady once said, "I prayed for this to happen but I didn't think it ever would."

Doubt cancels faith. James 1:6, *But let him ask in faith, with no doubting, for the one who doubts is like a wave of the sea that is driven and tossed by the wind. For that person must not suppose that he will receive any-thing from the Lord;*

Confidence is gained by doing something right and repeating it over and over. The home maker gains confidence when she makes a cake and the family tells her how good is taste. She has the confidence to do it again.

The brick mason begins by laying the bricks very carefully; tapping it just right to fit the line. With experience he can shove the brick in place.

Weigh yourself once each week. If your goal is to lose 20 lbs. you should lose two lbs. each week. The first week when you accomplish your goal you will have the enthusiasm to work harder the next week. As you lose the enthusiasm will continue with the accomplishments each week.

Suggestion: Never, Never, ever criticize anyone for anything. You may say, "How do people learn if you don't criticize their faults?" The words you speak can make or break an individual. Compliment their good points and they will discover their faults on their own.

Confidence can be gained from an imaginary event. This can be done by sitting in a comfortable chair and making your body relaxed. After becoming totally relax imagine doing something that you previously dreaded or was afraid to do. Imagine yourself doing the thing that you fear perfectly. Spend time to really get the feel of doing it without fear.

Practice this over and over. Remember anything you do constantly for 21 days will become a habit.

The other way this can be done is with hypnotism.

An young lady came to our class who wanted to be a pro Golfer. Her brother was the pro of a country club and she wanted to be as good as he was. I got her in a deep state of relaxation and instructed her to play nine holes of golf.

She followed my instructions. Every stroke was perfect in her imagination. After a few weeks she told me that she lowered her handicap 12 points. I played with her after she improved and she was great.

When we trust God with our self-confidence, we put the power in His hands. That can be scary and beautiful all at the same time. We've all been hurt and crushed by others, but God doesn't do that. He knows we aren't perfect, but loves us anyway. We can feel confident in ourselves, because God is confident in us. We may seem ordinary, but God never sees us that way. We can find our self-confidence safe in His hands.

So, how do we apply this to achieving our

goals. Our confidence is in God (not ourselves) that He will helps us to reach our goals.

Demand what you feel you deserve. Avoid giving in because of a lack of confidence.

The story was told that someone wanted Donald Trump to make a speech at a special venue in Central Park in NY City. He called and asked to speak to Mr. Trump. The secretary asked the nature of the call. He explained what he wanted and he was willing to pay $10,000.00. She replied, "I would not bother to relate the message for that amount. He said, "Maybe I could go $25,000.00." She said, "You are wasting your time he does make speeches for that amount."

Later he called back and said, "I have managed to raise $100,000.00 for Mr. Trump to make the speech." She said, "I will tell him, but I doubt that he will be interested. When she told trump about all the phone calls he said, "This guy is interesting. I will call him."

When trump called him, he quickly told him that he would not waste his time making a speech for $100,000.00. Trump told him, "the people won't be coming for any reason but to hear me." The man was insistent that he need him to make the speech. The two negotiated and Trump finally agreed to make the speech for $2,000,000.00. Later the man said it was worth every penny.

Just announced on news today, CNN is carrying the presidential debate. Commercials that normally cost $5,000.00 have been raised to $200,000.00 because of Trump's popularity.

Chapter Eight

Lend a Hand to Others

The Doll

I was walking around in a Wal-Mart store, when I saw a Cashier hand this little boy some money back. The boy couldn't have been more than 5 or 6 years old. The Cashier said, "I'm sorry, but you don't have enough money to buy this doll." Then the little boy turned to the old woman next to him, "Granny, are you sure I don't have enough money?" The old lady replied: "You know that you don't have enough money to buy this doll, my dear." Then she asked him to stay there for just 5 minutes while she went to look around. She left quickly.

The little boy was still holding the doll in his

hand. Finally, I walked toward him and I asked him who he wished to give this doll to. "It's the doll that my sister loved most and wanted so much for Christmas. She was sure that Santa Claus would bring it to her." I replied to him that maybe Santa Claus would bring it to her after all, and not to worry. But he replied to me sadly. "No, Santa Claus can't bring it to her where she is now. I have to give the doll to my mommy so that she can give it to my sister when she goes there."

His eyes were so sad while saying this… "My Sister has gone to be with God. Daddy says that Mommy is going to see God very soon too, so I thought that she could take the doll with her to give it to my sister." My heart nearly stopped. The little boy looked up at me and said: "I told daddy to tell mommy not to go yet. I need her to wait until I come back from the mall.'

Then he showed me a very nice photo of himself. He was laughing. He then told me 'I want mommy to take my picture with her so she won't forget me.'

"I love my mommy and I wish she didn't have to leave me, but daddy says that she has to go to be with my little sister." Then he looked again at the doll with sad eyes, very quietly.

I quickly reached for my wallet and said to the boy. "Suppose we check again, just in case you do have enough money for the doll!" OK' he said, 'I hope I do have enough." I added some of my money to his without him seeing and we started to count it. There was enough for the doll and even some spare money. The little boy said: "Thank you God for giving me enough money!"

Then he looked at me and added, 'I asked last night before I went to sleep for God to make sure I had enough money to buy this doll, so that mommy could give it to my sister. He heard me!" "I also wanted to have enough money to buy a white rose for my mommy, but I didn't dare to ask God for too much. But He gave me enough to buy the doll and a white rose." "My mommy loves white roses."

A few minutes later, the old lady returned and I left with my basket. I finished my shopping in a totally different state of mind from when I started. I couldn't get the little boy out of my mind.

Then I remembered a local news paper article two days ago, which mentioned a drunk man in a truck, who hit a car occupied by a young woman and a little girl. The little girl died right away, and the mother was left in a critical state. The family had to decide whether to pull the plug on the life-sustaining machine, because the young woman would not be able to recover from the coma. Was this the family of the little boy?

Two days after this encounter with the little boy, I read in the news paper that the young woman had passed away. I couldn't stop myself as I bought a bunch of white roses and I went to the funeral home where the body of the young woman was for people to see and make last wishes before her burial. She was there, in her coffin, holding a beautiful white rose in her hand with the photo of the little boy and the doll placed over her chest.

I left the place, teary-eyed, feeling that my life had been changed forever. The love that the little boy had for his mother and his sister is still, to this day, hard to imagine. And in a fraction of a second, a drunk driver had taken all this away from him.

Editors Note: This story has been around a while. I couldn't resist including it here. The rest of the stories are true.

The Good Samaritan

A long-time friend, Anita Morton, and her daughter were on a busy highway in a business area. She noticed that a policeman had stopped to assist a lady who was having car trouble.

After leaving the scene, she stopped at a drive-in restaurant for quick lunch. While paying her bill she noticed the same policeman was at the drive-in window. She told the clerk, "I'll pay for the policeman's lunch also."

She acknowledged that she saw the good deed he did for the lady in trouble and wanted to do something for him.

The Grocery Store

Some time ago, I was shopping for groceries at a local super market. While standing in the check-out line, I noticed that the lady in front of me tried to pay with a credit card and it was rejected. Then she wrote a check and the clerk couldn't accept it. She started to cry. I noticed what was in her basket and obviously there were children at home. She told the clerk, "I don't know what I am going to do."

I stepped in and told the clerk to put her groceries on my bill. Since she had already checked it through the register, she said, "Sir her bill is $55.00." I paid the clerk for her bill so she could leave. She graciously thanked me and left.

The Flower Bouquet

I was in a super market buying my wife flowers for Valentine's Day. I choose a nice bouquet of roses and went to the checkout counter. The clerk admired the flowers and said; "In my many years of marriage no one has ever brought me flowers."

As I walked to my car I couldn't get those words out of my mind. This senior lady longed for flowers and no one ever brought them.

I put the flower in my car and went back into the store. I told the lady who was arranging the flowers I wanted another bouquet exactly like the one I just bought. I gave her enough money to pay for the flowers and asked her to take them over to the clerk after I leave.

I never saw this clerk again, but I felt good for what I had done.

Sent By An Angel

I saw a lady standing by her car with a gas can in her hand. Obviously she was out of gas. I stopped and asked if I could help. She said. "I ran out of gas. I have a can, but I was afraid to leave my car."

I took her can and went to a nearby gas station and filled it. I brought it back to her car and poured it into the tank. She started the car, got out and asked how much she owed me. "You don't owe me anything," I told her. She said, "At least let me pay for the gas." I told her that wouldn't be necessary.

As I started to leave, I gave her a business card with Silent Angels on it. She said, I prayed for God to send someone, but I didn't have any idea He would send an Angel.

Silent Angels

In 1991, my wife and I formed Silent Angels Nonprofit. Our first mission was to distribute blankets to the homeless and disaster victims. I grew quickly to helping many categories of help in need. Below are some of our projects.

Firemen in Florida

Anita Daugherty Morton was instrumental in many fundraising projects. One was held at the K-Mart store in Spartanburg, SC. Tables were placed at the front door of the store to take collections and distribute literature. This event was dedicated to the firemen in Florida. Forest fires had gotten out of hand and were spreading fast. The firemen were exhausted and suffering from certain needs, medical and personal. This was probably the best fund-raiser we ever promoted (at this point). A total of $17,000.00 in cash and merchandise was collected. Many people asked what we needed and went into the store to buy the merchandise and brought it to our tables.

This event drew many volunteers including the Childs, Moores, Daughertys, DeZern and Smith families along with several others. Anita and her daughter, Cari accompanied Pat and Lorie Childs in delivering the merchandise and money to the firemen in Florida.

We later learned that the money was used to help purchase new equipment for the fire fighters.

New Furnishings for Home

My son-in-law, Robin Moore, who is a contractor, was asked to remodel a house in a poor neighborhood. After inspection, he told the rehab authorities that he would take the job, providing all the contents could be destroyed. They agreed. When the house was ready for the family to reoccupy, Silent Angels replaced all the furniture in the house.

Serving Disaster Victims

Other projects such as carrying water to hurricane victims in North Carolina and Georgia were headed by Donna and Robin Moore. The Moores also took a lead role in distributing blankets to the homeless in Washington, DC, We spent two days in DC with two pick-up trucks, two trailers and a van loaded with blankets, food and clothing. Arrangements had been made with Martha's Kitchen, a non-profit that feeds the homeless, to follow their vans and after the hungry people on the street ate their soup, they could get a blanket and clothes to take with them. This was a humbling experience for all who made the trip.

An interesting thing happened on the trip to Washington. We gave some clothes to many of the homeless. One man brought back the clothes we gave him. He said, "I can't take these." We asked, "Why?" He said, "At night I sleep in a tree and the police will spot me wearing white clothes."

In February 1998, we heard on the news that a tornado touched down in Kissimmee, Florida and an entire sub-division was leveled. Johnnie and I drove to the blanket manufacturer we were dealing with and bought a truck load of blankets and headed to Florida. After surveying the damage, we went to the Kissimmee Church of Christ and where a headquarters was set up to distribute clothing, food and blankets. Before we could unload people were standing in line to receive a blanket.

On one occasion, as we often do, we parked at a The Second Presbyterian Church Soup Kitchen to distribute blankets. We were struck by passion when we heard a man, holding a blanket close to his chest say, "Look guys, see what I got, this is just what I needed."

Will Work For Medicine

Sometimes we tend to pass by beggars on the street holding signs, "Will work for food." I observed a man standing between the lanes of a busy highway holding a sign, "Will work for medicine." I stop and got his attention. He told me his story, "My wife and I were visiting in North Carolina and she had an allergic reaction to some washing powder at a coin laundry. She stayed in the hospital three days.

When she was released, the doctor gave her three prescriptions and we don't have the money to get them filled." I asked him to get in my car and we drove to the nearest pharmacy. He gave the prescriptions to the clerk and asked what the cost would be. While they were filling getting the medication ready he pulled some money out of his pocket and said, this is what I have collected today." It was $43.00. I took his money and waited for the prescriptions to be filled. I carried him back to his car where his wife was waiting. As I told him goodbye, I gave the $43.00 back to him and said, "You need this to buy gas."

On one occasion, a couple of our grandchildren asked, "How do you know they will use the money for food and not alcohol?" My wife, Johnnie, replied, "It is our responsibility to help them. It is their responsibility to spend the money wisely.

Helping Dangerous Communities

My daughter, Donna, arranged an event for Silent Angels in cooperation with two religious groups. The event was to give blankets, food and heating fuel to a poor community. The event was held in a well known drug community. For about thirty minutes we drove through the community, with someone yelling from the car, "Blankets, food and kerosene." We set up a space with the blankets. A church group cooked and served a meal. Another group had 55 gallon drums of kerosene with a dispensing spout. Soon people were coming from behind buildings, down the railroad, and from all directions. We were warned several times to be careful because of the nature and habits of the people. It was a good day. Many people were helped with no incidents.

Special Angels

"Special Angels" are children with some type of disability. During the years of Silent Angels, I had taken special interest in a little girl I met at the age of one. Megan Warren has a muscular disability. At this writing she is 14 and I still see or hear from her occasionally. We continue to add Special Angels to our list.

Tsunami Relief

When the Tsunami hit Asia in 2004, we organized a drive to collect food clothing and etc. My wife, Fran, did most of the organizing for the event, which was most successful. We had donations from many churches, schools, businesses and individuals.

There was one hitch during the campaign. After collecting all the food, we were informed it would be a waste of time and expense to ship it, because in that particular area, they do not eat the food we collected. The food was distributed through local homeless services.

Most of the donations went to India.

Gospel Partners

Gospel Partners is a group in America, founded by Ray Brinkley to help support orphans and widows in India. After his death his son and daughters continue the work their father started. The government has ordered that the orphans and the widows be housed separately. A fund fundraising is being done to pay for the land and construction of the home for the orphans, which has already been started. It is urgent that funds be raised to meet the needs.

A group of children were brought to the

school in 2008 after their parents died in the 2004 tsunami that devastated much of south Asia. The children lived in a fishing village on the Bay of Bengal. They were with care takers in a hostel while their parents were out in their fishing boats when the tsunami struck. 25 children woke up to the horrible news that their parents were dead. I cannot imagine the fear and overwhelming sadness that the children were cared for by minister Joshiraju of the church of Christ after their parent's death. However, there is only land but no church building there. Therefore, the children lived mainly in the open on the beach for 4 years until Bro. Joshiraju asked bro Jayaraju take the children to Tanuku to live and go to school at Brinkley Memorial School. Before bro. Jaya knew about the children one child died leaving 24 children. After the decision was made to bring the children to Tanuku 2 little brothers lay down in the sea grasses and died in the night. Jaya and Joshiraju bought boxes and buried the boys.

The following week 22 children were brought to Tanuku by the staff of Brinkley School...each staff member gave $5.00 of their small salaries to help transport the children to the school. The children were cleaned and checked by a doctor and were given 3 nutritious meals a day. In a few months they looked like different children.

Silent Angels continue to work with Gospel Partners to help the orphans.

Homeless in Zagreb, Croatia

I met a missionary from Croatia and became interested in his work. Silent Angels made several donations to help the homeless in his country. Part of the money was used to purchase and washer and dryer which they placed in the church building. This allowed the homeless to come in and wash and dry their clothes.

Part of the donations were use to print a large

number of tracts to distribute throughout the city of Zagreb, which had a population of more than one million.

Hurricane Katrina

When hurricane Katrina hit the Gulf Coast in 2005, Donna and Robin Moore organized a mission trip to Mississippi. They carried two trucks and two trailers with medical supplies, blankets and other needs to the victims. Along with it they carried a crew of five with a Bob Cat tractor, chain saws and other equipment.

In March 2006, another mission trip was planned. The Central Church of Christ in Spartanburg collected items for care packets including wash clothes, soap, shampoo, hand lotion, toothbrushes and toothpaste. The members packaged these items in gallon-size plastic bags and prepared them for shipment. We also had a large amount of freeze-dried foods donated which were left from the Y2K scare of 2000. Toby McCall organized a work group of nine men, which included himself, Tommy McCall, Al Smith, Tim Fagan, Dave Long Jon Hall, Jeff Perry, Robert Dickerson and me.

We delivered the goods to the Carrollton Avenue Church of Christ in New Orleans. We got our assignment, which was to build two separate rooms in a flooded school building and install 16 shower stalls. In eight days we completed our assignment, including all the electrical and plumbing. The project also included restoring electricity throughout the entire first floor of the building. Tommy McCall, being an electrical contractor, did an admirable job with the assistance of Robert Dickerson.

New Orleans was unbelievably destroyed. Some of the crew had served in military overseas remarked, "This is worse than any war zone I witnessed in service."

We all were physically exhausted but mentally we felt good that the job was completed. Since then hundreds have slept in the school and the showers we built.

Silent Angels of OZ

From 1980 to 1988, I worked with the late Raymond Brinkley of Orlando Florida, to promote and raise funds for his mission work in India. Many times I wanted to go with him, but circumstances prevented me from going.

As I wrote newsletters, I could visualize what it would be like, as a missionary in India.

My interest in mission work started in the middle 60s. When I wrote a newsletter for a missionary in Africa.

In 2005, David French came to our church and talked about mission work in Zambia. Although, his primary interest was teaching and spreading the Kingdom of God in Zambia, he mentioned that aids is taking the lives of so many people and leaving behind thousands of orphans. He stated that, they have an interest in caring for orphans, but time and finances would not allow it at this time.

At this time we were involved in the New Orleans project, which was taking all our energy.

With this mission behind us, I was looking for a new opportunity. I remembered the plight of the orphans in Zambia. All during this time the orphans kept coming to my mind. Frequently, I went to the internet to learn more about Zambia and the number of orphans that were roaming the streets.

We gave some thought to going back to New Orleans, but the orphans in Zambia seemed like the next outreach for us.

Without discussing the idea with David French, I boldly announced during a bible class that I wanted Silent Angels to raise $100.000.00 to build an orphans home in Zambia. The announcement came as a surprise to many. The numbers seemed unreachable to others. Then, others volunteered to go and help.

I contacted David, by email and told him what our plans were. He informed me of the pros and cons of such a project. First, a board of directors from Zambia would have to be formed to get permission from the government. Then, they would have to find suitable property for the home and make arrangements to lease it. No real estate is privately owned in Zambia. The government owns all of it. Individuals and groups actually lease the land.

About a year later, David, his wife Lorie and their daughter Natasha came for another visit. He explained that his work with Mapepe Bible College was full-time and he didn't have the time to organize an orphans program, but he has appointed Richard Waggoner from Tennessee, to direct the program.

I asked for Richard's email address and contacted him. Within a few weeks, Richard and his wife came to the Central Church of Christ in Spartanburg to tell us about his plans for the orphans program.

Richard explained that this would not be the average type of orphans home, because with so many orphans in Zambia, we could never make a dent in housing orphans.

The orphans care would be a temporary facility for homeless children, until they could be placed in foster care. Richard was already managing a program where orphans were being placed in homes of widows. Richard and others were raising funds to pay for the food, clothing, education and medical for these youngsters.

Richard proposed that Silent Angels form an outreach called Silent Angels of OZ (orphans of Zambia.) I presented this idea to our Board and it was enthusiastically approved. In 2008, we organized "Silent Angels of OZ,"

With the cooperation of Richard and Ruth Orr, we raise $100,000.00.

In March 2009, I accompanied Richard Waggoner on a trip to Lusaka, Zambia. Our plans were to start construction on the house, but unfortunately, the rains were not over.

While there we spent most of our time visiting orphans who are being cared for by widows in the area. Food, clothing and medical care is being provided to about 200 orphans. Thomas Sakala, a native of Zambia, is in charge of administering the program.

The house was built under the supervision of David French. Orphans to occupy this home will come from prison. They were arrested for stealing food because they were hungry. Often when the parents die, the grandparents will put the children on a bus to Lusaka with a one-way ticket. They wonder around to the point of starvation, and then they steal food. This home will offer rehabilitation to these youngsters ages 7 to 17, who were living on the streets with no place to go.

David and Lorie French's daughter Karen, takes in babies whose mothers died at child birth and no one would accept responsibility for caring for the child. The law is that when a mother dies during child birth and no one claims the baby, the baby is thrown into the grave with the mother and buried alive. She expects to take in at least 10 babies.

Wide-Wide World To Serve

Silent Angels has now become a world-wide organization! Here is a partial list of recipients:

- Blankets for the homeless, food, clothing, furniture, shelter and medical needs, across the USA & parts of the world.
- Tornado & Hurricane Victims
- Equipment for firefighters
- Handicapped Children (Special Angels)
- Children's homes: Southeastern Children's

Home, Children's Home in India, Widows Children's Home, Kakinada, India, Children's Home, Chennai, India

- Homeless in Zagreb, Croatia
- Transportation: Honduras
- Palmetto Bible Camp
- Gospel Partners
- Tsunami victims in Asia
- Personal Care Packets for homeless shelters
- Relief supplies for victims of Katrina.
- Personal & medical items sent to Zambia.
- Assisted with "Operation Nehemiah" to help re-build New Orleans.
- St. Luke Free Medical Clinic
- Second Presbyterian Soup Kitchen

Today we continue to help support the orphans in India (Gospel Partners) and in Zambia (Silent Angels of OZ).

Helping others brings good feelings to the giver

and the receiver of the good deeds. Using your special gifts to help others can be a gift to yourself as you enjoy a self esteem boost for making others' lives better, and make the world a better place. You feel more worthy of good deeds yourself, your trust in the decency of people is reinforced, and you feel more connected to yourself and to others.

What does all this have to do with weight loss?

Think of ways that you can help others. Encourage them such as tell them how well they look, encourage them to stay on their diet, exercise and take their pill regularly.

Form a small group where you and your friends can meet weekly and discuss the progress of every one.

Chapter Nine

Learn to Accept Disappointments

Life is not always perfect. Things go wrong. Plans are sometimes interrupted. Earlier we said, "Life is filled with ups and downs. Your attitude when you are down will determine how high you will go when you are up."

Pam Stone is an actress, comedian, writer, and talk radio host. She played Judy Watkins in the 1990s television show "Coach."

She received a call recently from Hollywood saying that they were making a sequel to coach and wanted all the original cast so they could pickup where the show ended. NBC had paid for the show to be done and it was scheduled to air February

2016.

The cast were excited. They all went to Hollywood except one who choose not to be in the new show. They rehearsed four days and on the fifth day they filmed the pilot. The writer was not pleased with everything; he wanted to do a re-write. They were sent home for a few days while the re-write was being done.

A few days later, they got a call saying that NBC had canceled the show. WOW! What a disappointment.

Pam got the call while she was out of town having dinner with Mary Wilson of the Supremes. It was a shock. When she flew back home and saw the beauty of her farm with flowers planted by her wonderful husband; She says that she is okay with the decision.

What a gracious attitude! That's what makes her such a wonderful person.

Here are four steps that will help you to deal

with disappointments. (Copied from the Internet by Raeeka a yoga instructor.)

1. Let it out. One of the hardest things to do in a world where everything is immediate — we are all under external pressure, and time is a scarce resource — is to just let yourself experience a feeling.

Even at the most difficulties times, such as grieving, on average we only allow ourselves 1 to 2 weeks off or work, and then we mostly expect to get back into normality again.

Human beings are not very good at allowing the experiencing of emotions in full without trying to speed up the process. The only time we have this ability in its purest sense is when we are young children who have yet to be told or taught what is socially acceptable.

Children will tantrum and cry and scream, or laugh until it runs out and they are genuinely ready to move on.

I'm not suggesting we lock ourselves away for

weeks at a time whenever we have been disappointed, but to be aware of any sense of obligation to "just get over it."

Allow yourself to feel what you're feeling without any agenda of speeding up the process. Whatever you are feeling is OK. Take some time to just sit with your emotion and experience it without moving to fix or change it.

Genuinely experiencing emotions, no matter how painful, is one of the beauties of life. Don't shy away from these moments. Be present in them.

2. Get some perspective. The wonderful thing about letting it out is that you have given yourself that time. You have said to yourself, "I care about you. I want to allow you to feel what you need to feel and I do not wish to push you or cajole you."

You have treated yourself like a friend and allowed yourself the space you needed to experience your feelings of disappointment.

Once you've done that, it becomes much easier to get some perspective. After you give yourself space to feel, you're able to give the situation or individuals involved more room to breathe.

Perhaps the person who you feel disappointed by doesn't even realize they've done something to upset you. Maybe they're stressed out and don't have the emotional bandwidth to think about it because they aren't allowing themselves time to experience their emotions.

Giving yourself space to be as you are prepares you to allow the same to other people.

Having a broader perspective than your own view on a particular situation is always helpful. The critical point here is that you have to mean it. Rushing onto gaining perspective before you've allowed yourself to be with how you feel will be artificial and will not last.

3. Know your own heart. Disappointment can ripple through to the core of who you are. If you don't know what your core values are, you may not have a framework to support you when you experience negative emotions.

For example, one of my core values is open-heartedness. I wish to keep an open heart and be ready to share love and kindness with others, irrespective of how they might behave.

I would like to always try to choose to act with love and kindness towards others, rather than with negativity.

When someone disappoints me and I feel like closing and withdrawing, I remember this core value, then pause and make a choice.

I wish to be an open-hearted person. These negative feelings are feelings, and they will pass. Do I choose to remain open-hearted, or do I choose to follow the easier instinct and close off?

More often than not, I choose to be in line

with my values over the automatic response to the situation. It doesn't happen every single time, but most.

Knowing your own heart and your values gives you the freedom of choice. You can choose to be driven by what happens to you, or you can choose to live in line with your principles.

The latter has helped me to overcome disappointments and negative situations in a healthy way. The challenge of disappointment allows me to practice living closer to my values, and stops me from being swallowed up by it.

4. Practice acceptance. As human beings, even though we know that some things are bound to happen, we're not always willing to accept them.

Every time I am disappointed, I feel overwhelmed by my emotions. I'm inclined to withdraw and blame others, wanting to wallow in my disappointment. Each time, I have to accept that I will feel these things again.

I have to accept that I will continue to be disappointed—that it is a part of life, part of being human. I also have to accept that I will probably continue to struggle to accept this fact, at various points throughout the rest of my life!

This step is a lifelong challenge and fundamental to dealing with disappointment. I will be disappointed, I will disappoint, you will be disappointed, and you will disappoint. Life will be disappointing—but it will pass.

Practice acceptance and we may suffer less as it is happening and notice the good things in life more.

Disappointment is a part of life, but all parts of life can help us grow. We can be present and aware even in the midst of negative emotions and therefore live more fully.

(Great advice)

The sooner we learn to roll with the punches the greater our chances are for reaching our goals.

When a pilot leaves an airport he is given a bearing to set his instruments. Along the way he will receive new readings because the winds have pushed the aircraft off course.

When you find yourself off course reset your mental instruments to adjust your course. For some reason you may have to reset your goal date; that's okay.

Chapter Ten
Persist with Unrelenting Force

No great achievement is possible

without persistent work.

Bertrand Russell

The most interesting thing about a postage

stamp is the persistence

with which it sticks to its job.

• Napoleon Hill

•

If you don't know where you are going,

you will probably end up somewhere else.

– Lawrence J. Peter

Years ago, I was listening to Paul Harvey on Radio.
He began his broadcast with a commentary on per-

sistence. He said, "For years I have studied the lives of successful people and the only difference I can find between a successful person and a failure is that the failures give up too soon."

Ways of developing persistence:

Before you can develop persistence and eventually achieve success, you need to first identify your wants or desires. You can do this by simply writing down specifically all the things you want to have or accomplish. List down all your desires and wants, no matter how impossible they are to achieve at the moment.

Motivation comes from a deep reason why we want to achieve or have something. If you know why you're doing what you're doing, it gives you more energy to keep moving.

For an instance, you want to publish a book. Creating a book takes time and patience. If you don't have enough motivation, a reason why you need to publish the book, you probably can never finish it. But if you're motivated by the thought of influencing and teaching millions of readers thru your words, only then will you keep pushing yourself to work on finishing the book.

Outline your definite action. Identifying your wants or desires speaks of what you want to achieve. Determining your motivation shows the reasons why you want to achieve what you want. Outlining your definite action step is necessary to know how you will be able to achieve what you want.

When you know how to get what you want, it makes it easier to achieve it. To know how, it pays to do some research and planning of what needs to be done on your part. Be specific on each step you need to take.

Keep a positive mental attitude. The road to success is not easy, in fact, it's challenging, this is why only few succeeds. There will be countless times you will be face with defeat and failures that if you are weak, you'll be giving in to negative thoughts of fears and doubts.

In order to develop persistence and eventually succeed in your endeavor, always maintain a positive mental attitude, regardless of situation. Keep your thoughts focused on taking action towards your goals. Avoid negative thoughts and feelings for it will ruin your concentration and persistence.

All your goal-setting and planning will go to waste if you won't be able to develop discipline and good habit. There will be a lot of hindrances that will stop you from moving towards your goal, and without proper discipline, it will be easy for you to sail away. Upholding discipline and good habits can help you stay in the course, even despite difficulties.

This story illustrates my point:

When Henry Ford was manufacturing the A - models back in the early 1900s a man created an automatic transmission. He carried it to Ford and wanted him to use them in his cars. Ford said, "I need to see it demonstrated."

The inventor set up a demonstration. He said, All you have to do is push this button and you are ready to go. But, just in case it doesn't work you push this button." Ford said, Hold on, I don't want a product that has doubts in it." He said, "Mr. Ford I know it will work the other button is just in case it doesn't work,." Ford said, "I don't want a just in case." He replied, "Mr. Ford you don't understand, "God knew a man couldn't have a baby, but He gave him two breast just in case."

Make sure all the flaws are addressed when making your plan for success.

There was a story of a plantation owner working at the grist mill. He didn't notice a sharecropper's little girl enter the door. He said, "Get out of here or I'll give you a beating you'll never forget." She took three steps forward and said, "My mama said send her fifty cents." With all the command he could he ordered her to get out. Then he went back to work She didn't move. She took three more step toward him. He picked up a stick and said, "I told you to get out." With a strong voice she said, "My mama's got to have that fifty cents." He paused a while and out his hand in his pocket and gave her the fifty cents. She left and he sat down on a box trying to conceive that he had been beaten by a little girl.

One of my favorite stories is a snail slowly climbing up a cherry tree. On the way to the top he met a beetle. "Where are you going?" the beetle asked. "I am going to the top of the tree to get some cherries," he answered. The beetle laughed and said, "This is winter time. There are no cherries up there." The snail said, "At my pace there will be by the time I get there."

One writer sent her manuscript to a publisher 37 times. On the 37th try it was accepted and she got an advance check for $100,000.00.

Remember this self-motivator. **"In any adversity I accept no defeat. I look for the seed of an equivalent or great benefit, and fight persistently toward my goal, thankful for the lesson I learned."**

Never, ever, give up and you will succeed.

Chapter Eleven

Kill Fears & Doubt

If fear and doubt are uncontrolled they can destroy your dreams. You have to kill them in their tracks.

If you are like most people, you have a goal or a dream that is meaningful and that you want to achieve. That goal may be related to personal growth issues such as weight loss, gaining self-esteem, finding inner peace, increasing your energy levels, or overcoming depression.

Or, your goal may include going back to school, entering a new career, or bringing your creative talents into a greater public light. Having a goal is the easy part. Attempting to move through your own inner obstacles can literally leave you terrified, completely paralyzed by your own fear.

Examples where fear kills your dreams:

- "I'd love to visit Africa, but what if something bad happens while I'm there? I'll go somewhere else instead."

- "I'd love to write a book, but what if people hate it? Maybe I should read more before I start writing."

- "I'd love to get in shape, but what if I look stupid at the gym? I need to lose some weight before I go."

Don't pick goals where the stakes are low.

When the gym owner chooses to avoid competition and only miss lifts in her home gym, it's a way of keeping the stakes low. But failing in a safe zone is just a clever way of holding yourself back.

If you fail inside your comfort zone, it's not really failure, it's just maintaining the status quo. If you never feel uncomfortable, then you're never trying anything new.

Nobody is rooting for you to fail. Maybe you'll succeed. Maybe you'll fail. For the most part, nobody cares one way or the other.

This is a good thing! The world is big and you are small, and that means you can chase your dreams with little worry for what people think.

Just because you don't like where you have to start from doesn't mean you shouldn't get started.

Feelings of fear and uncertainty have a way of making you feel unprepared.

"I should learn more before I take this test."

"I should practice more before I compete."

"I should get this degree before I start this business."

Here's a tough question that forces you to consider the opposite side: How long will you put off what you're capable of doing just to maintain what you're currently doing?

Stop making uncertain things, certain. Who says you're going to fail? Just because someone else got rejected from that job doesn't mean you will. Maybe the publisher hated your friend's book, but that doesn't mean they'll hate yours. Maybe you tried to lose weight before, but that doesn't mean you can't lose it now.

You're not destined to "miss that lift." In fact, maybe you're destined to succeed.

Stop acting like failure is certain. It's not.

The only real failure is not taking any action in the first place.

We all deal with feelings of fear, uncertainty, and vulnerability. And unfortunately, most of us let those feelings dictate our actions. For this reason, the simple decision to act is often enough to separate you from most people. You don't need to be great at what you do, you just need to be the one person who actually decides to do it.

You can enjoy a lot of success by doing the things that most people make excuses to avoid.

The greatest thing to fear is fear itself. Most of us were raised in a negative atmosphere. Our life started with don'ts.

Don't climb the tree you might fall.

Don't go swimming until you lean how.

Don't play with the cat, it might scratch you.

The list of don't go on and on.

A salesman walked you to the porch where a little girl was playing. What's your name he asked? "Suzie no no," she answered. Her name had been followed with no, no so many time she actually thought it was part of her name.

The Great Depression was caused by Fears and doubts. People thought the banks were going broke so they demanded their money. As a results many lost their life savings. The whole country was in a state of panic.

In 1974, There was a gas shortage. Again people panicked. Many gas stations were closed. Some only allowed a customer to buy a few gallons.

What caused the problem was fear and doubt. People were buying the minimum amount and getting in the back of the line to buy more. Without this fear the lines would have been much shorter.

There were fights at the gas pumps. Not only fights some were shot and killed.

Remember earlier we talked about the sub-conscious mind accepts everything we see, hear feel, touch and taste. It accepts everything as fact. It does not know any gray areas.

When you say "I am afraid I can't do it" the sub-conscious say, "He don't want to do it let's give him reason to be afraid."

"I'm afraid I will forget my speech." The sub-conscious says, "He does want to remember his speech let's help him to forget it."

That may sound too simple but, it is very true. Be careful what you say, what you read, what you listen to others say, do or what you are exposed to, your subconscious mind is listening.

Vita-Guard Weight Loss Formula

Vita-Guard Weight Loss Formula is a combination of carefully selected multiple vitamins and minerals. My wife, Johnnie and I were employed by a diet company to train doctors how to sell the weight loss product to their patients. With that background and my experience with other vitamin programs, I used my experience to help with this book.

To find a representative for Vita-Guard in your area, send me an email to: vitaguard1912@gmail.com. Or go to the website: Vita -Guard.com.

You may order directly by sending $29.95 plus $7.25 S&H to Vita-Guard, 91 E. Main Street, Inman, SC 29349.

Become a Vita-Guard Representative

Vita-Guard is a fast growing company that sells vitamins for a healthy body and a weight loss product that will help to produce Permanent Weight Loss.

The need for Vita-Guard is growing every day. You can become a representative and help to fill that need and earn a commission at the same time.

We pay 20% retail profit, expense account and retirement.

Send an email to: vitaguard1912@gmail.com

For more information.